STRETCHING EXERCISES FOR SENIORS OVER 60

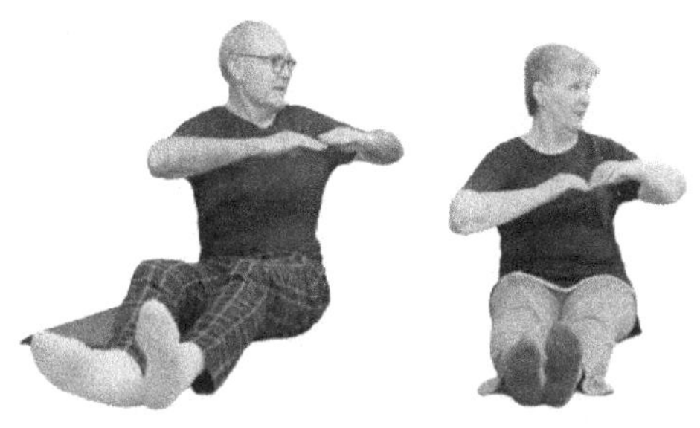

Easy Workouts to Enhance Flexibility, Alleviate Stiffness, Ease Pain, through Strength Training for active seniors over 60

James Stewart

CONTENTS

"Stretching is a simple
and beneficial activity
that can improve your
health and well-being.
All you need is a
comfortable space,
some basic knowledge,
and a positive
attitude."

INTRODUCTION

As we age, our bodies undergo many changes that affect our mobility, flexibility, and overall quality of life. Our muscles tend to lose strength and elasticity, our joints become stiffer and less lubricated, and our posture and balance may deteriorate. These changes can make us more prone to injuries, chronic pain, and reduced functionality in our daily activities.

However, there is a simple and effective way to counteract these effects of aging and maintain or even improve our physical and mental well-being: stretching. Stretching is the act of elongating or extending a muscle or a group of muscles to increase their range of motion and flexibility. Stretching can have many benefits for seniors, such as:

- Enhancing blood flow and oxygen supply to muscles and organs.

- Reducing muscle tension and stiffness
- Enhancing joint mobility and lubrication

- Preventing or relieving back pain, neck pain, and other common musculoskeletal problems

- Increasing coordination and balance

- Boosting energy and mood

- Promoting relaxation and stress relief.

- Supporting healthy aging and longevity

Stretching can also complement other forms of physical activity, such as walking, swimming, or yoga, by preparing the body for movement and preventing injuries. Stretching can also be done as a standalone activity, at any time and place, with minimal or no equipment. All you need is a comfortable space, some basic knowledge, and a positive attitude.

In this book, you will learn everything you need to know about stretching for seniors, including:

- How to stretch safely and effectively

- The best time and frequency to stretch

- The anatomy and physiology of stretching

- The different types of stretching

- Avoiding common errors in stretching and ensuring proper technique

- A 10-minute warm-up routine

- A 10-minute cool-down routine

- Over 65 stretching exercises for the whole body, with clear illustrations and step-by-step instructions.

- How to customize your stretching routine based on your fitness level, health condition, and personal preferences.

- How to incorporate stretching into your daily activities, such as gardening, walking, or household chores.

- How to use props, such as a chair, a wall, a towel, or a resistance band, to enhance your stretching experience
- How to deal with common challenges or obstacles that seniors may face when starting or maintaining a stretching habit, such as motivation, boredom, pain, or injury.

-Measuring your advancements and commemorating your accomplishments.

By following the guidance and tips in this book, you will be able to enjoy the many benefits of stretching and improve your quality of life. Whether you are new to stretching or have some experience, this book will help you make stretching a fun and rewarding part of your daily routine. So, what are you waiting for? Let's get started!.

CHAPTER 1:

How to Stretch Safely and
Effectively

Stretching is a simple and beneficial activity that can improve your health and well-being. However, like any other form of exercise, stretching requires some basic knowledge and precautions to avoid injury and maximize results. In this chapter, you will learn how to stretch safely and effectively, by following these guidelines:

- Consult your doctor before starting a stretching program, especially if you have any medical conditions, injuries, or chronic pain. Your doctor can advise you on the best types and intensity of stretching for your situation, and warn you about any potential risks or contraindications.

Warm up before stretching, by doing some light cardio or dynamic movements for 5 to 10 minutes. This will increase your blood flow, raise your body temperature, and prepare your muscles and joints for stretching. Warming up can also prevent muscle strains and tears, and enhance your performance and flexibility.

- Stretch gently and gradually, by applying a mild and comfortable tension to the target muscle or muscle group. Do not bounce, jerk, or force your stretch, as this can cause damage to your tissues and trigger a protective reflex that tightens your muscles. Instead, hold your stretch for 15 to 30 seconds, and breathe deeply and slowly. You should feel a slight pull or discomfort, but not pain. If you feel pain, stop immediately and adjust your position or intensity.

Stretch both sides of your body equally, by performing the same stretch on the opposite side. This will help you maintain a balanced and symmetrical posture and alignment, and prevent muscle imbalances and injuries. Try to keep your body as aligned and stable as possible, and avoid twisting or bending your spine excessively.

- Stretch after your main activity, by doing some static or passive stretches for 10 to 15 minutes. This will help you cool down, relax your muscles, and improve your recovery. Stretching after your activity can also prevent muscle soreness and stiffness, and increase your range of motion and flexibility over time.

Stretch regularly and consistently, by making stretching a part of your daily routine. The more you stretch, the more benefits you will reap. Aim to stretch at least 3 times a week, preferably every day, and vary your stretches to target different muscles and joints. You can also stretch at different times of the day, such as in the morning, during breaks, or before bed, to suit your schedule and preferences.

- Listen to your body and be mindful of your sensations, by paying attention to how you feel before, during, and after stretching. Your body will give you feedback and signals that can help you adjust your stretching program to your needs and goals. For example, if you feel tight or stiff, you may need to stretch more or longer. If you feel sore or injured, you may need to rest or modify your stretches. If you feel relaxed and refreshed, you are doing it right.

By following these guidelines, you will be able to stretch safely and effectively, and enjoy the many benefits of stretching for seniors. Remember, stretching is not a competition or a chore, but a way to enhance your health and happiness. So, have fun, be gentle, and keep stretching!.

1.1 The Anatomy and Physiology of Stretching

To understand how stretching works and why it is beneficial, it is helpful to have some basic knowledge of the anatomy and physiology of stretching. Anatomy is the study of the structure and shape of the body and its parts, while physiology is the study of how the body and its parts function and interact. In this chapter, you will learn about the main components and processes involved in stretching, such as:

- The skeletal system, which consists of the bones and joints that provide support and structure to the body. The skeletal system also allows movement and protects the internal organs. There are different types of joints in the body, such as hinge joints (e.g., elbow and knee), ball-and-socket joints (e.g., shoulder and hip), and gliding joints (e.g., wrist and ankle). Each joint has a different range of motion, which is the degree of movement that a joint can perform in different directions.

The muscular system, which consists of the muscles and tendons that attach to the bones and enable movement and force. The muscular system also maintains posture and generates heat. There are different types of muscles in the body, such as skeletal muscles (e.g., biceps and quadriceps), cardiac muscle (e.g., heart), and smooth muscles (e.g., stomach and intestines). Each muscle has a different function, structure, and innervation, which is the connection to the nervous system.

- The nervous system, which consists of the brain, spinal cord, and nerves that control and coordinate the body's activities. The nervous system also receives and processes sensory information from the environment and the body. There are different types of nerves in the body, such as sensory nerves (e.g., touch and pain), motor nerves (e.g., movement and reflexes), and autonomic nerves (e.g., digestion and heartbeat). Each nerve has a different role, origin, and destination.

The stretch reflex, which is a protective mechanism that prevents excessive stretching of a muscle and its associated structures. The stretch reflex is triggered when a muscle is stretched beyond its normal length, causing a contraction of the same muscle and a relaxation of the opposite muscle. The stretch reflex involves a sensory receptor called the muscle spindle, which detects changes in muscle length and tension, and a motor neuron, which transmits the signal to the muscle fibers. The stretch reflex can be overridden by the brain, which can inhibit or enhance the reflex depending on the situation.

- The length-tension relationship, which is the relationship between the length of a muscle and the force it can produce. The length-tension relationship is influenced by the arrangement and overlap of the muscle fibers, which are composed of smaller units called sarcomeres. The sarcomeres contain two types of protein filaments, called actin and myosin, which slide past each other to cause muscle contraction and relaxation. The optimal length of a muscle is the length at which it can generate the most force, which is usually around its resting length. When a muscle is too short or too long, it cannot produce as much force, and its performance and efficiency are reduced.

The flexibility, which is the ability to move a joint or a group of joints through their full range of motion. Flexibility is influenced by many factors, such as age, gender, genetics, activity level, injury history, and muscle temperature. Flexibility can be improved by stretching, which increases the length and elasticity of the muscles and other connective tissues, such as ligaments and fascia. Stretching can also improve the lubrication and nutrition of the joints, and reduce the stiffness and adhesions of the tissues.

By learning about the anatomy and physiology of stretching, you will be able to appreciate the complexity and beauty of the human body, and how stretching can enhance its function and health. You will also be able to apply this knowledge to your stretching practice, by choosing the best types and methods of stretching for your goals and needs. In the next page, you will learn about the different types of stretching, and their advantages and disadvantages.

1.2 The Different Types of Stretching

Stretching is not a one-size-fits-all activity. There are different types of stretching, each with its own purpose, technique, and effect. In this chapter, you will learn about the main types of stretching, and how to choose and perform them correctly. The main types of stretching are:

Static stretching:

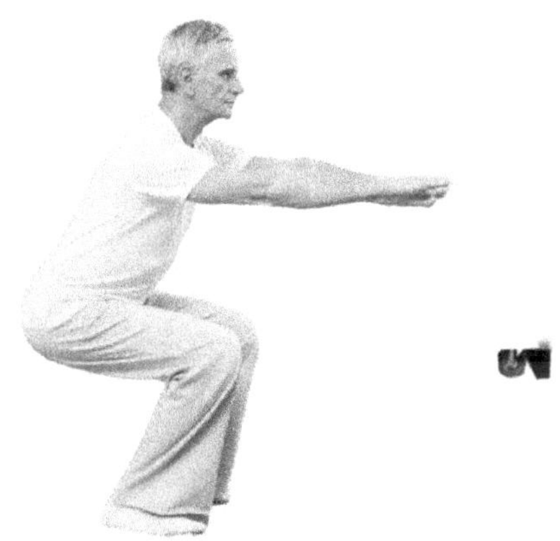

This is the most common and familiar type of stretching. Static stretching involves holding a stretch position for a certain amount of time, usually 15 to 30 seconds, without moving or bouncing. Static stretching can improve your flexibility and range of motion, and reduce muscle tension and soreness. Static stretching is best done after your main activity, when your muscles are warm and relaxed, or as a separate activity, such as before bed or in the morning. Static stretching can also be done before your main activity, but only after a proper warm-up, and with a lower intensity and duration, to avoid reducing your muscle strength and power.

Dynamic stretching:

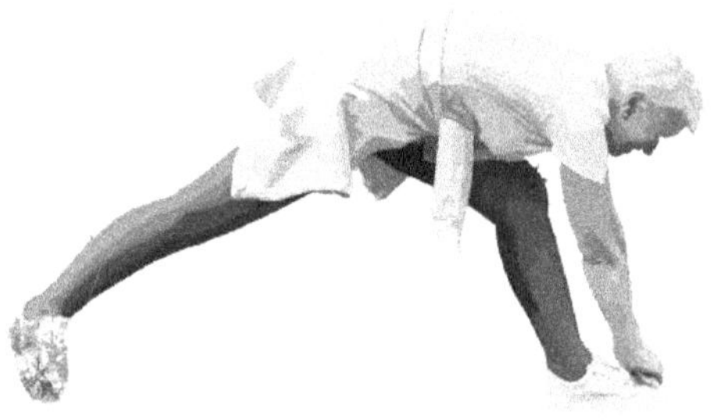

This is a type of stretching that involves moving your joints and muscles through their full range of motion, with controlled and fluid movements. Dynamic stretching can improve your blood circulation, muscle temperature, joint lubrication, and coordination. Dynamic stretching is best done before your main activity, as part of your warm-up, to prepare your body for movement and prevent injuries. Dynamic stretching can also be done after your main activity, as part of your cool-down, to restore your normal range of motion and prevent stiffness.

Passive stretching:

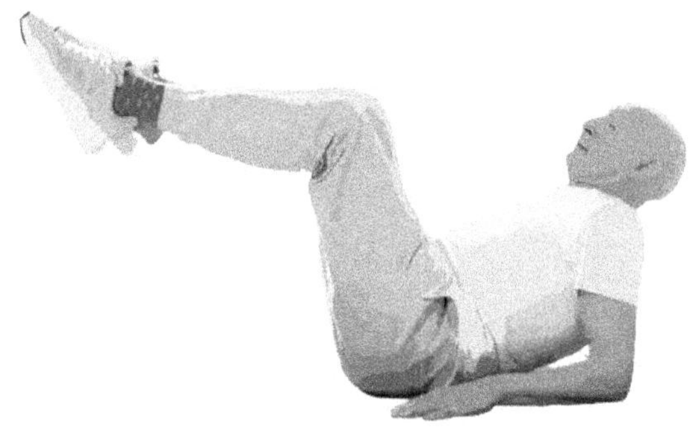

It is a type of stretching that involves using an external force, such as a partner, a prop, or gravity, to assist or enhance your stretch. Passive stretching can increase your flexibility and range of motion, and relax your muscles and mind. Passive stretching is best done after your main activity, when your muscles are warm and relaxed, or as a separate activity, such as before bed or in the morning. Passive stretching can also be done before your main activity, but only after a proper warm-up, and with a lower intensity and duration, to avoid reducing your muscle strength and power.

Active stretching:

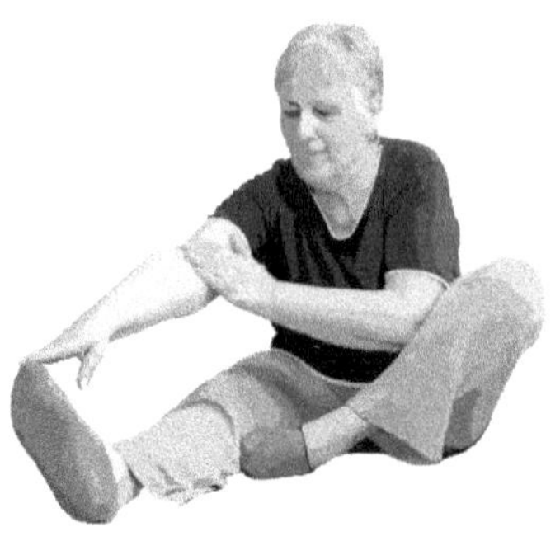

which is a type of stretching that involves contracting the opposite muscle or muscle group of the one being stretched, to create a tension that pulls the target muscle into a stretch. Active stretching can improve your flexibility and range of motion, and strengthen your muscles and joints. Active stretching is best done before your main activity, as part of your warm-up, to prepare your body for movement and prevent injuries. Active stretching can also be done after your main activity, as part of your cool-down, to restore your normal range of motion and prevent stiffness.

These are the main types of stretching, but there are also other types, such as ballistic stretching, isometric stretching, proprioceptive neuromuscular facilitation (PNF) stretching, and yoga, which are variations or combinations of the above types. Each type of stretching has its own advantages and disadvantages, and you should choose the type that suits your goals, needs, and preferences. You can also mix and match different types of stretching, depending on the situation and the body part you want to stretch. In the next chapter, you will learn about the most common stretching mistakes and how to avoid them.

"Stretching can improve your blood circulation, joint mobility, posture, balance, energy, mood, relaxation, and longevity. What more can you ask for?"

CHAPTER 2:

The Most Common Stretching Mistakes and How to Avoid Them

Stretching is a simple and beneficial activity that can improve your health and well-being. However, if done incorrectly, stretching can also cause harm and hinder your progress. In this chapter, you will learn about the most common stretching mistakes and how to avoid them, by following these tips:

Do not skip the warm-up or the cool-down. Warming up and cooling down are essential parts of any physical activity, including stretching. Warming up prepares your body for movement and prevents injuries, while cooling down restores your normal range of motion and prevents stiffness. To warm up, do some light cardio or dynamic movements for 5 to 10 minutes. To cool down, do some static or passive stretches for 10 to 15 minutes.

Do not stretch too hard or too long. Stretching should be gentle and gradual, not painful or excessive. Stretching too hard or too long can damage your tissues and trigger a protective reflex that tightens your muscles. Instead, stretch to the point of mild discomfort, but not pain, and hold your stretch for 15 to 30 seconds, depending on your goal and preference. You can repeat the same stretch 2 to 4 times, or switch to a different stretch, but do not overdo it.

<u>Do not hold your breath or tense your body.</u> Breathing and relaxing are important aspects of stretching, as they help you release tension and increase your flexibility. Holding your breath or tensing your body can have the opposite effect, as they can cause stress and reduce your range of motion. Instead, breathe deeply and slowly, and relax your body as much as possible. You can also use visualization or meditation techniques to enhance your relaxation and focus.

<u>Do not neglect your posture or alignment.</u> Posture and alignment are crucial for stretching, as they affect the quality and effectiveness of your stretch. Neglecting your posture or alignment can lead to improper stretching, which can cause muscle imbalances and injuries. Instead, pay attention to your posture and alignment, and keep your body as stable and symmetrical as possible. You can also use a mirror, a partner, or a video to check your form and correct any errors.

__Do not forget to vary your stretches and target different muscles and joints__. Stretching the same way every time can lead to boredom and plateau, which can reduce your motivation and results. Forgetting to stretch some muscles or joints can also lead to tightness and weakness, which can affect your performance and function. Instead, vary your stretches and target different muscles and joints, depending on your goals, needs, and preferences. You can also try different types of stretching, such as static, dynamic, passive, or active, to spice up your routine and challenge your body.

By avoiding these common stretching mistakes, you will be able to stretch safely and effectively, and enjoy the many benefits of stretching for seniors.

2.1 A 10-Minute Warm-Up Routine

A warm-up is an essential part of any physical activity, including stretching. A warm-up prepares your body for movement and prevents injuries, by increasing your blood flow, raising your body temperature, and enhancing your joint mobility and lubrication. A warm-up can also improve your performance and flexibility, by activating your muscles and nervous system, and reducing your muscle tension and stiffness.

A warm-up should be done before your main activity, such as walking, swimming, or yoga, or before your stretching session, if you are doing it as a separate activity. A warm-up should last for about 10 minutes, and consist of two phases: a general warm-up and a specific warm-up.

A general warm-up is the first phase of a warm-up, and it involves doing some light cardio or aerobic exercises, such as jogging, cycling, skipping, or jumping jacks. The purpose of a general warm-up is to increase your heart rate and blood circulation, and to warm up your whole body. A general warm-up should last for about 5 minutes, and be done at a low to moderate intensity, depending on your fitness level and preference. You should not feel exhausted or out of breath, but rather slightly sweaty and energized.

A specific warm-up is the second phase of a warm-up, and it involves doing some dynamic or active stretches, which are stretches that involve moving your joints and muscles through their full range of motion, with controlled and fluid movements. The purpose of a specific warm-up is to target the specific muscles and joints that you will use in your main activity or your stretching session, and to prepare them for movement and force. A specific warm-up should last for about 5 minutes, and consist of 10 to 15 different dynamic or active stretches, depending on your goals and needs. You should not feel pain or discomfort, but rather a slight pull or challenge.

Here is an example of a 10-minute warm-up routine, that you can follow or modify to suit your situation and preference:

General warm-up (5 minutes): Jog for 5 minutes at a comfortable pace, or choose another light cardio or aerobic exercise that you enjoy.

Specific warm-up (5 minutes): Perform the following dynamic or active stretches, each for 30 seconds, with a 10-second rest in between. You can repeat the same stretch on both sides, or switch to a different stretch, depending on your body part and preference.

Neck rolls: Slowly rotate your head in a circular motion, clockwise and counterclockwise, to loosen up your neck and shoulders.

Shoulder circles: Lift your shoulders up to your ears, then roll them back and down, in a circular motion, clockwise and counterclockwise, to warm up your shoulder joints and muscles.

Arm swings: Swing your arms forward and backward, across your chest and behind your back, to stretch your chest and upper back muscles.

Torso twists: Stand with your feet shoulder-width apart, and your arms extended to the sides. Slowly twist your torso to the right and left, keeping your hips and legs stable, to stretch your lower back and oblique muscles.

Hip circles: Stand with your feet shoulder-width apart, and your hands on your hips. Slowly rotate your hips in a circular motion, clockwise and counterclockwise, to lubricate your hip joints and muscles.

Leg swings: Stand with your feet hip-width apart, and your hands on a wall or a chair for balance. Swing your right leg forward and backward, as high as you can, to stretch your hamstrings and hip flexors. Repeat with your left leg.

Knee lifts: Stand with your feet hip-width apart, and your arms by your sides. Lift your right knee up to your chest, and hug it with your hands. Release and switch to your left knee. Alternate between your right and left knees, to stretch your quads and hip flexors.

Ankle rolls: Stand with your feet hip-width apart, and your hands on a wall or a chair for balance. Lift your right foot off the ground, and rotate your ankle in a circular motion, clockwise and counterclockwise, to warm up your ankle joint and muscles. Repeat with your left foot.

By following this 10-minute warm-up routine, or a similar one, you will be able to prepare your body for your main activity or your stretching session, and prevent injuries and enhance your results. Remember, a warm-up is not optional, but mandatory, for any physical activity, including stretching. So, do not skip it, and enjoy it!

CHAPTER 3

Stretching Exercises for the Neck and Shoulders.

1. Neck Tilts:

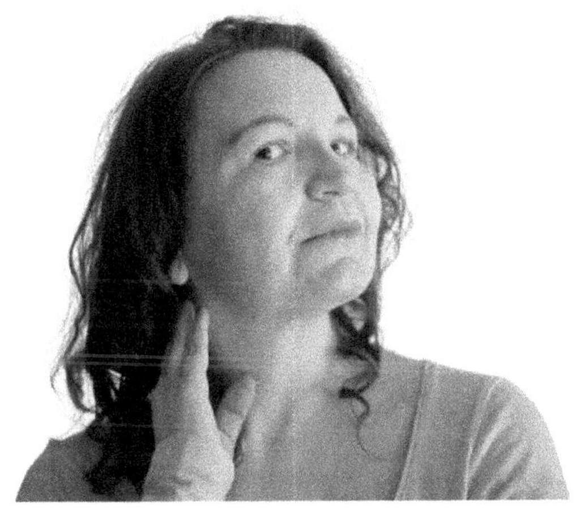

- Find a comfortable sitting or standing position.

- Slowly incline your head to one side, bringing your ear toward the shoulder.

- Maintain the stretch for 15-30 seconds.

- Repeat the process on the opposite side.

2. *Neck Rotation*:

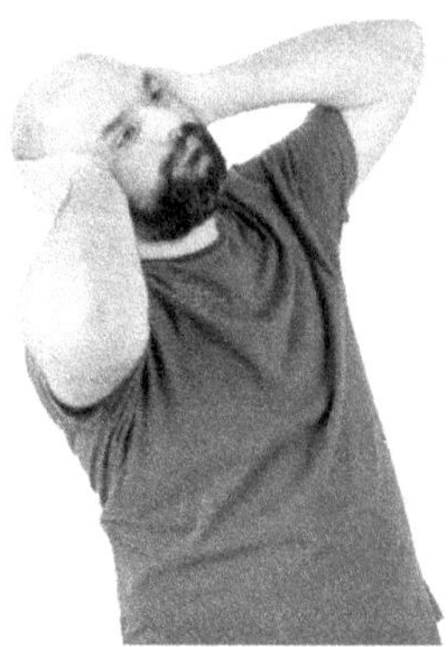

- Gently turn your head to one side, bringing your chin over the shoulder.

- Hold the stretch for 15-30 seconds.

- Repeat the movement on the other side.

3. *Neck Flexion:*

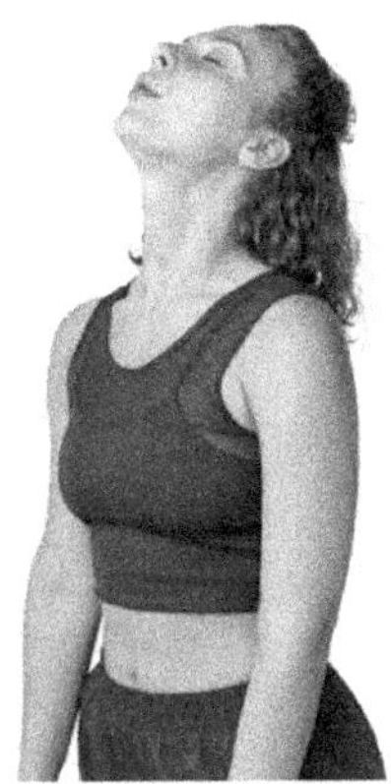

- Gradually lower your chin towards your chest.

- Hold the stretch for 15-30 seconds.

4. **_Shoulder Rolls:_**

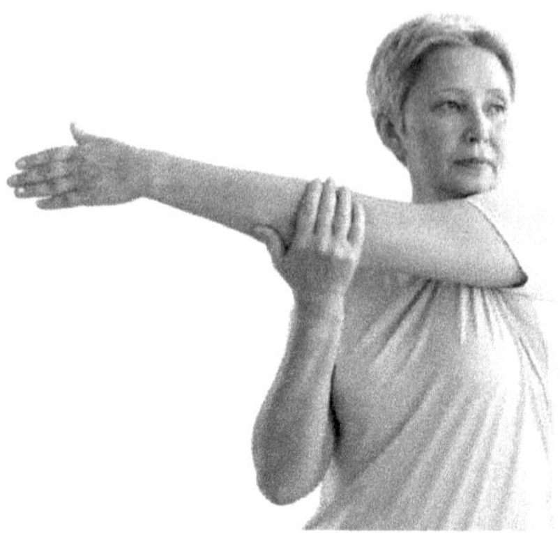

- Rotate your shoulders backward in a circular motion.

- Complete 10-15 rotations.

- Change direction and roll your shoulders forward.

5. *Shoulder Stretch:*

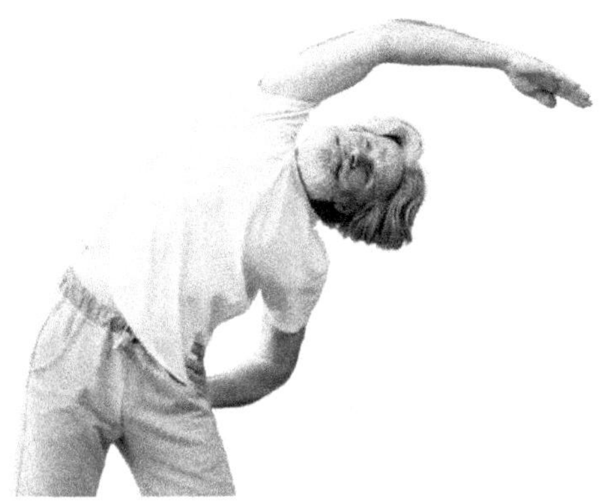

- Extend your right arm across the chest.

- Use your left hand to gently press the right arm toward the chest.

- Hold for 15-30 seconds.

- Repeat the stretch on the opposite side.

6. *Neck and Shoulder Stretch*:

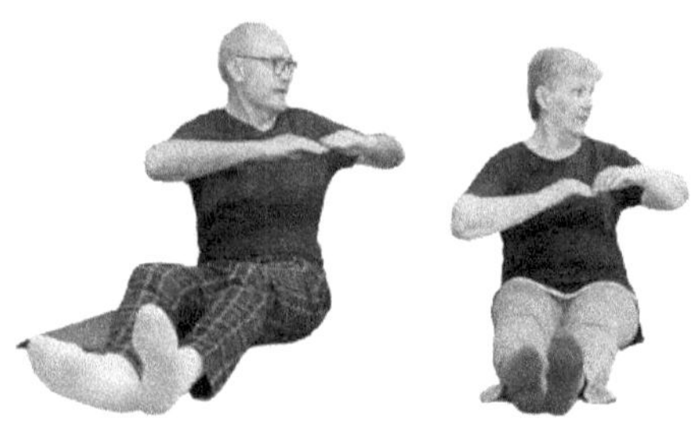

- Interlock your fingers and extend your arms in front.

- Round your back and bring your chin towards the chest.

- Feel the stretch in the neck and shoulders.

- Maintain for 15-30 seconds.

Always perform these stretches with a slow and gentle approach, avoiding any movements that cause pain. Consult a healthcare professional if you encounter discomfort.

3.2 Stretching Exercises for the Upper Back and Chest

1. Neck and Shoulder Rolls:

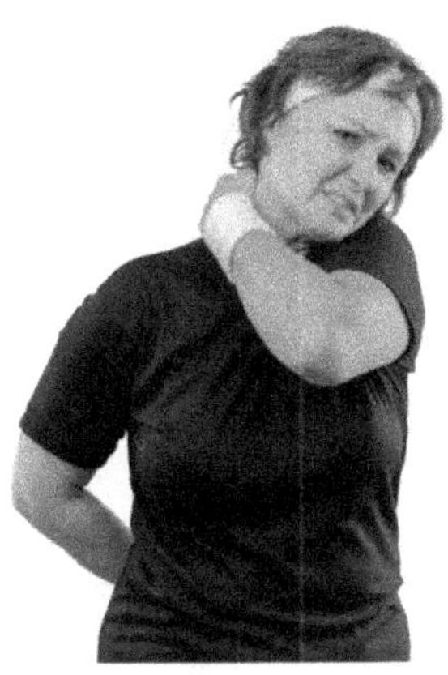

- Begin by sitting or standing in a comfortable position.

- Roll your shoulders backward and forward gently.

- Incorporate neck rolls, moving your head side to side.

2. *Chest Opener Stretch*:

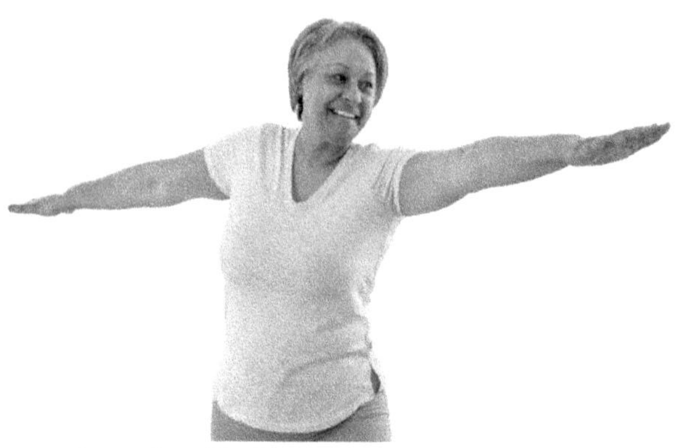

- Stand tall, keeping your feet hip-width apart.

- Clasp your hands behind your back, extending your arms.

- Elevate your chest, creating a gentle stretch across the front of your body.

3. *Wall Angels*:

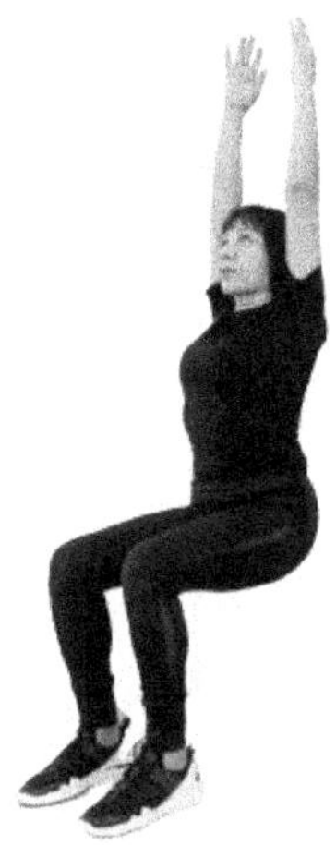

- Position yourself with your back against a wall.

- Raise your arms to shoulder height, pressing them against the wall.

- Gradually slide your arms upward and then back down, mimicking snow angels.

4. *Doorway Stretch*:

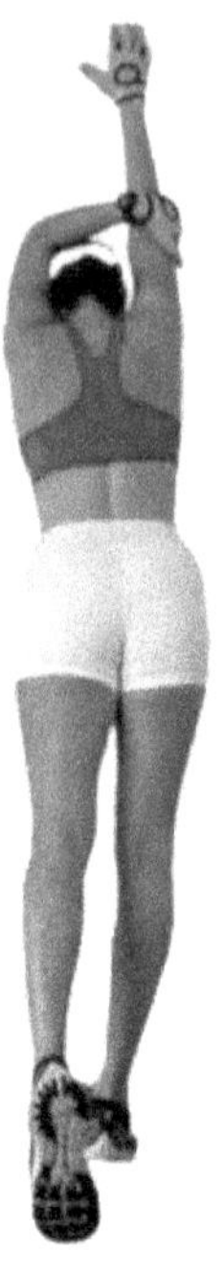

- Stand within a doorway with arms bent at a 90-degree angle.

- Lean gently forward, experiencing the stretch in your chest and upper back.

5. *Child's Pose*:

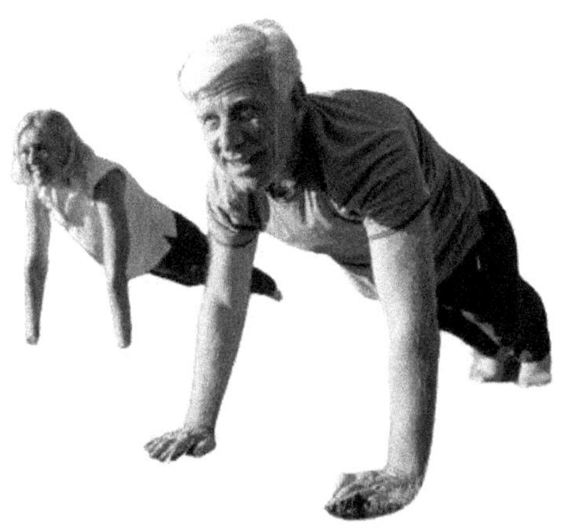

- Commence on hands and knees.

- Sit back onto your heels, extending your arms forward on the floor.
- Relax your chest towards the ground.

6. *Seated Twist*:

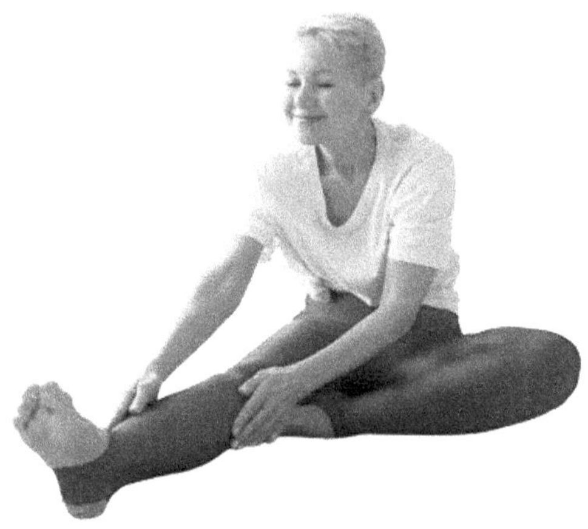

- Sit cross-legged or with legs extended.

- Twist your torso to one side, using the opposite arm to deepen the stretch.

- Switch sides.

7. *Cat-Cow Stretch:*

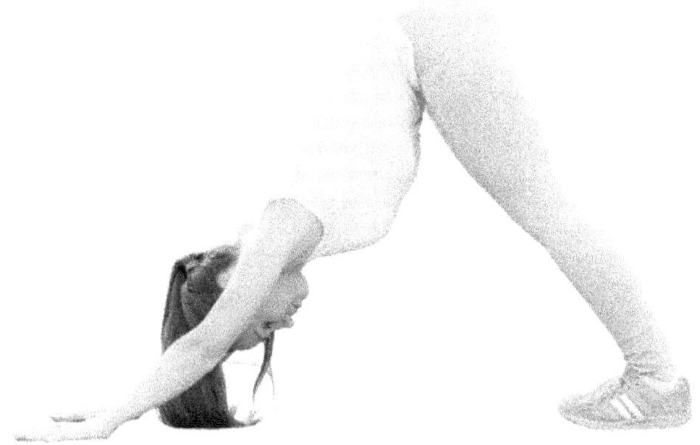

- Start on your hands and knees.

- Arch your back upward (cat position) and then lower it down (cow position).

- Repeat to enhance spine flexibility.

Always perform these stretches with care and pay attention to your body. If you experience any discomfort, discontinue the exercise. Consulting with a healthcare professional before initiating a new exercise routine, especially for seniors, is recommended.

3.3 Stretching Exercises for the Arms and Hands guide:

1. **Wrist Flexor Stretch**:

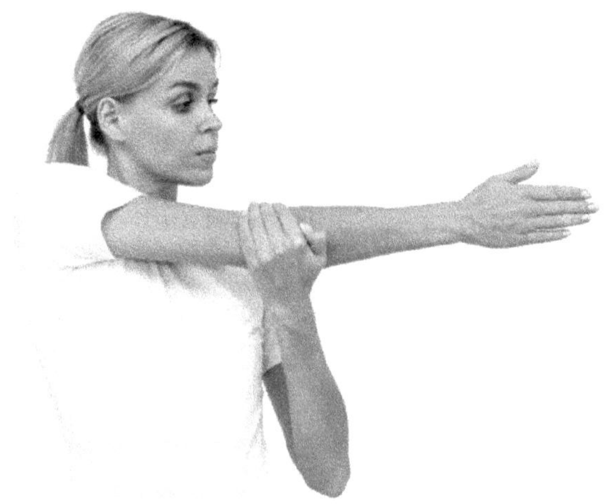

- Sit or stand comfortably.

- Extend your right arm, palm facing down.

- Gently press down on your right hand with your left hand.

- Hold for 15-30 seconds.

- Repeat on the opposite arm.

2. *Triceps Stretch*:

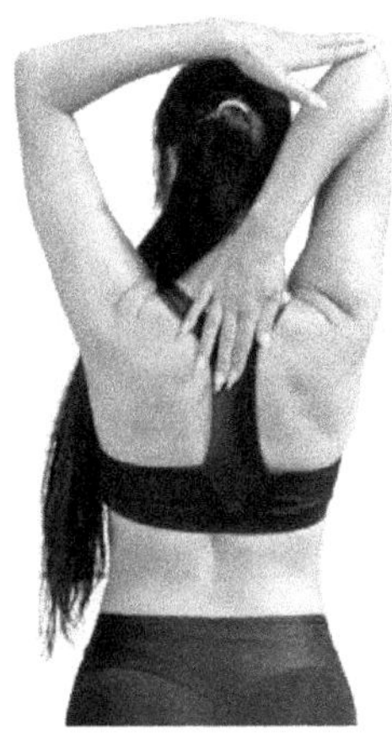

- Lift your right arm and bend it, bringing your hand down your back.

- Use your left hand to gently push on your right elbow.
- Hold for 15-30 seconds.

- Repeat on the other arm.

3. ***Bicep Stretch***:

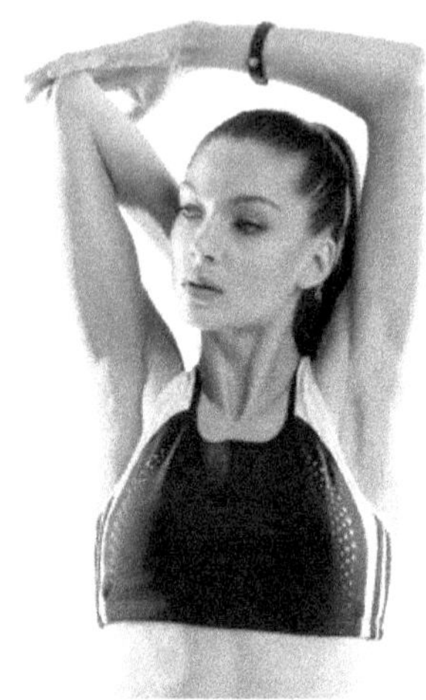

- Straighten your right arm, rotating the palm to face up.

- Bend the arm at the elbow, using your left hand to pull your fingers toward your shoulder.

- Hold for 15-30 seconds.
- Repeat on the opposite arm.

4. *Forearm Stretch*:

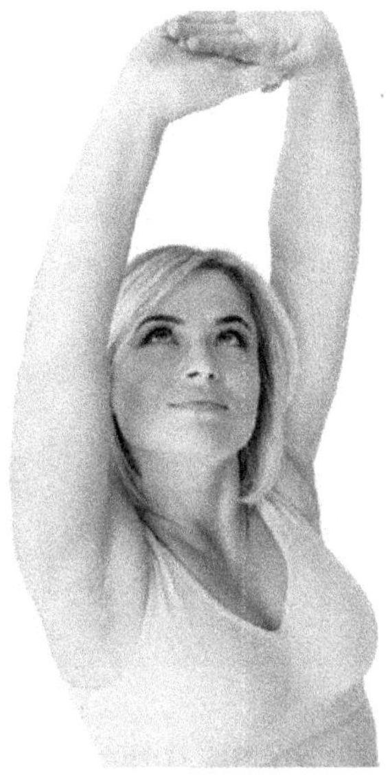

- Extend your right arm in front.

- Point your fingers down, and use your left hand to gently press on the back of your right hand.

- Hold for 15-30 seconds.
- Repeat on the other arm.

5. *Finger Stretch*:

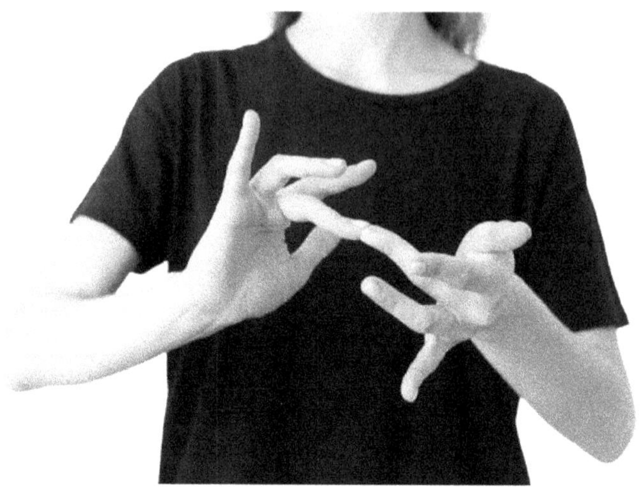

- Interlock your fingers in front of you.

- Press and straighten your arms while keeping fingers interlocked.

- Hold for 15-30 seconds.

6. ***Thumb Stretch***:

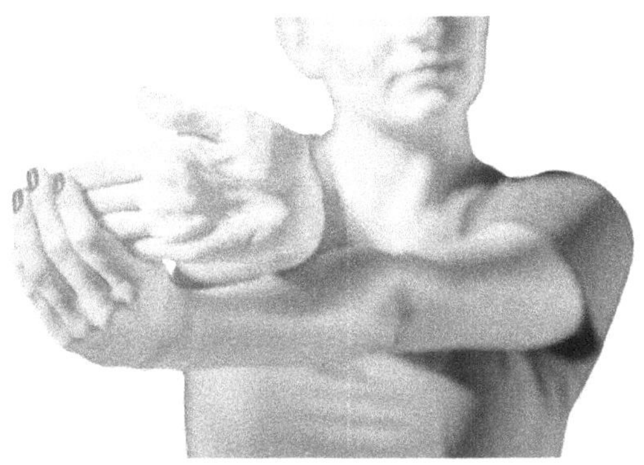

- Hold your right hand in a fist.

- Gently extend your thumb away from the fingers.

- Hold for 15-30 seconds.
- Repeat on the other hand.

Perform these stretches slowly, avoiding bouncing, and hold each stretch to a point of mild tension. Adjust the intensity based on your comfort. Always consult a healthcare professional before starting new exercises, especially for seniors.

3.4 Stretching Exercises for the Lower Back and Hips

1. **Warm-Up**:

- Initiate your routine with a mild warm-up, such as a light stroll or cycling, to boost blood circulation to your muscles.

2. **Seated Forward Bend**:

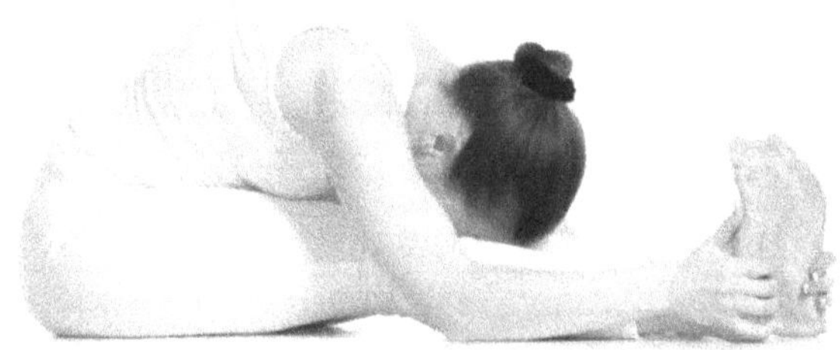

- Position yourself on the floor with legs extended.

- Gently lean forward at the hips, reaching towards your toes.

- Maintain the stretch for 15-30 seconds, sensing the stretch in your lower back and hamstrings.

3. **Cat-Cow Stretch**:

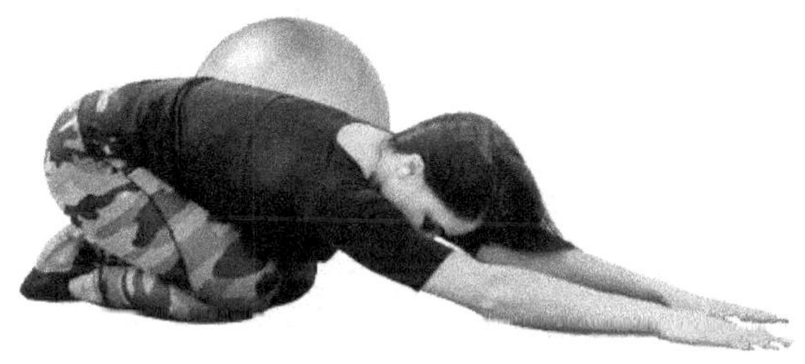

- Commence in a tabletop position on hands and knees.

- Arch your back upward (cat) and then lower it down (cow) in a fluid sequence.

- Repeat for 1-2 minutes to enhance spinal flexibility.

4. *Child's Pose stretch*:

- Kneel on the floor, sit back on your heels, and extend your arms forward.

- Lower your chest to the floor, experiencing a gentle stretch in your lower back.

5. **Hip Flexor Stretch**:

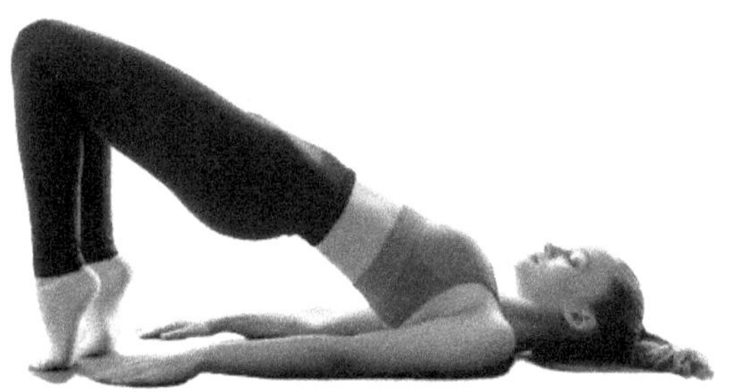

- Kneel on your right knee with the left foot in front, creating a 90-degree angle.

- Shift your weight forward, extending the front of the right hip.

- Maintain the position for 15-30 seconds, then switch sides.

6. *Piriformis Stretch*:

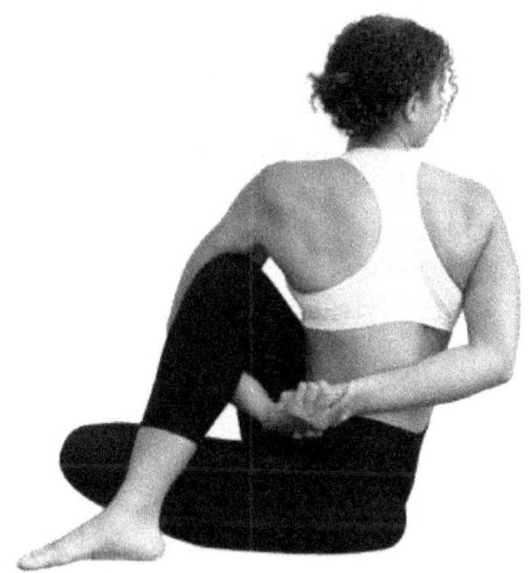

- Sit with one leg crossed over the other.
- Embrace your knee and delicately rotate towards the crossed leg.

- Hold for 15-30 seconds, feeling the stretch in the outer hip.

7. **_Knee-to-Chest Stretch_**:

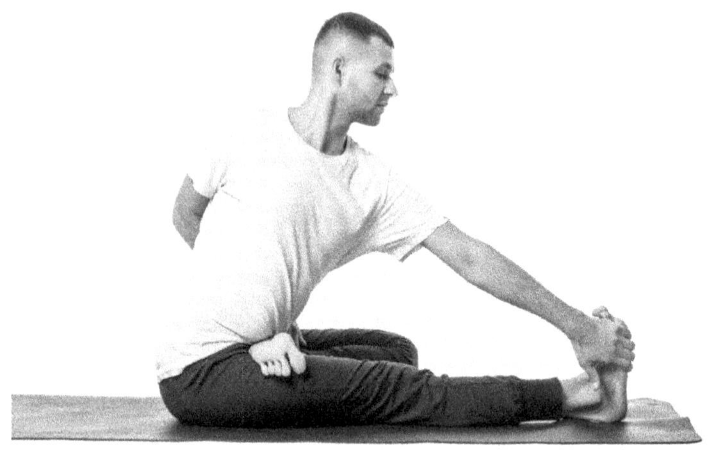

- Recline on your back, draw one knee towards your chest, and clasp it with both hands.

- Hold for 15-30 seconds, then alternate legs.

8. *Supine Spinal Twist*:

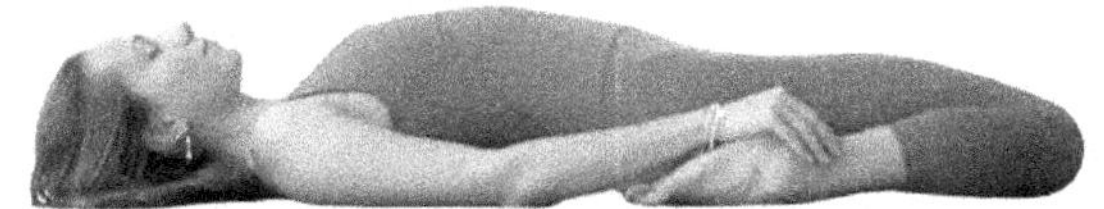

- Lie on your back, bring one knee across your body, with the opposite shoulder grounded.

- Maintain the position for 15-30 seconds, then swap sides.

9. **_Bridge Exercise_**:

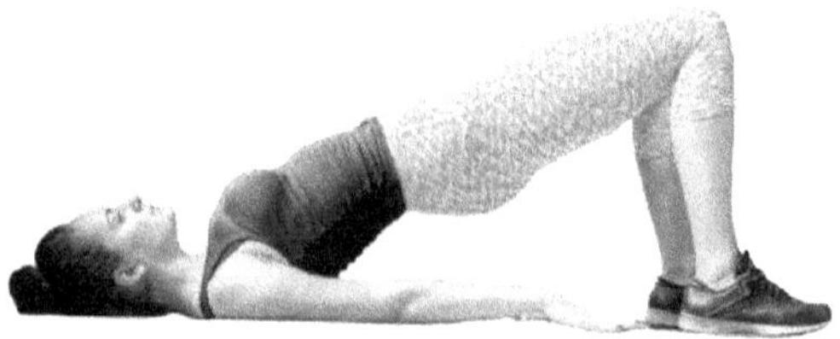

- Lie on your back, bend your knees, and elevate your hips towards the ceiling.

- Hold for a few seconds, activating your glutes and lower back muscles.

10. *Cool Down stretch*:

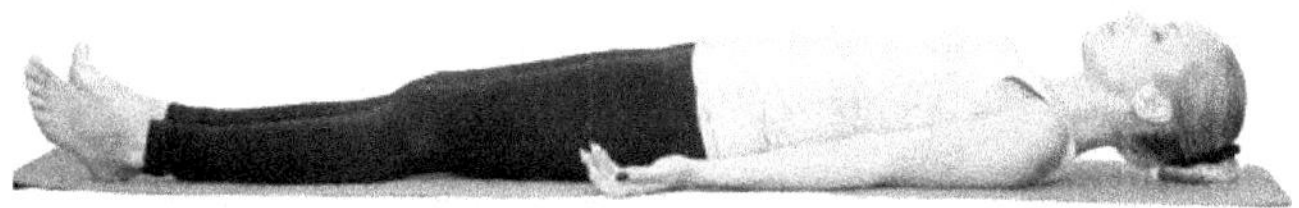

- Conclude your routine with gentle stretches or relaxation exercises for a gradual cool down.

Remember to heed your body's signals, and if any stretch induces discomfort, ease off. Integrate these exercises slowly into your regimen for enhanced flexibility and well-being in your lower back and hips.

3.5 Stretching Exercises for the Legs and Feet guide

1. Warm-up:

- Initiate your routine with a mild warm-up, engaging in light cardio activities such as five minutes of walking in place to enhance blood circulation to your legs and feet.

2. Ankle Circles:

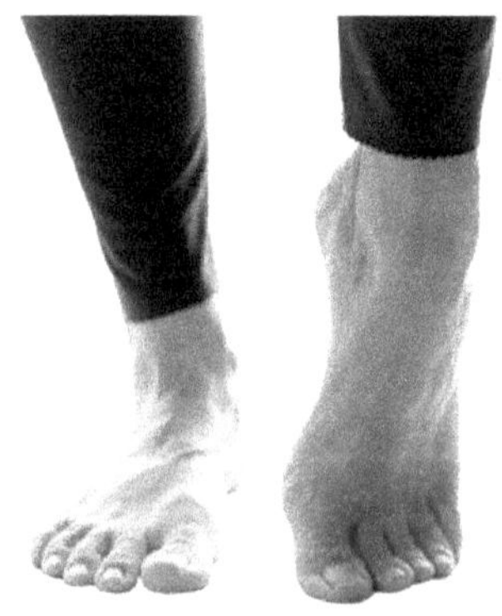

- Whether seated or standing, raise one foot and rotate the ankle clockwise and then counterclockwise.

- Repeat this motion ten times before switching to the opposite foot.

3. *Toe Flexor Stretch:*

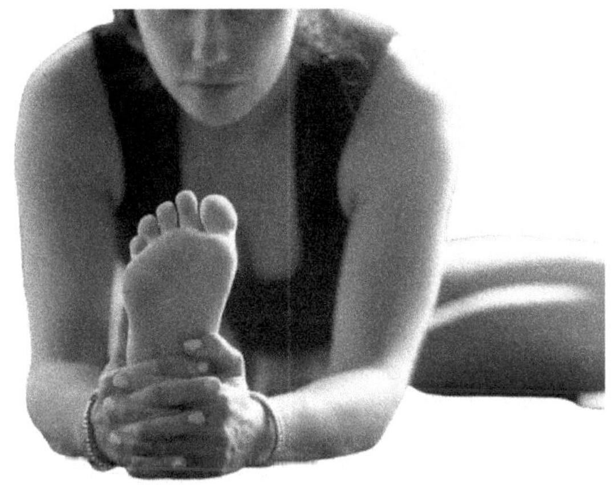

- Seated with legs extended, point and flex your toes alternately, holding each position for ten seconds.

- repeating the sequence multiple times.

4. **Calf Stretch**:

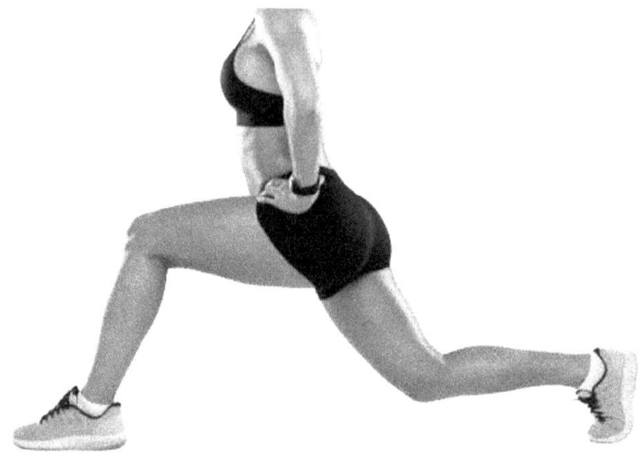

- Stand facing a wall, place hands on it, and step one foot back straight, bending the front knee.

- Maintain this position for 15-30 seconds before alternating to the other foot.

5. *Quadriceps Stretch:*

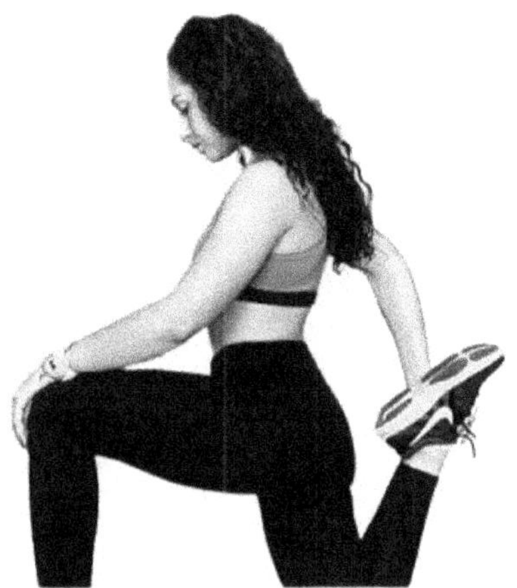

- While standing, raise one foot toward your buttocks, grasping the ankle with your hand.

- Hold for 15-30 seconds and then switch to the other leg.

6. *Hamstring Stretch*:

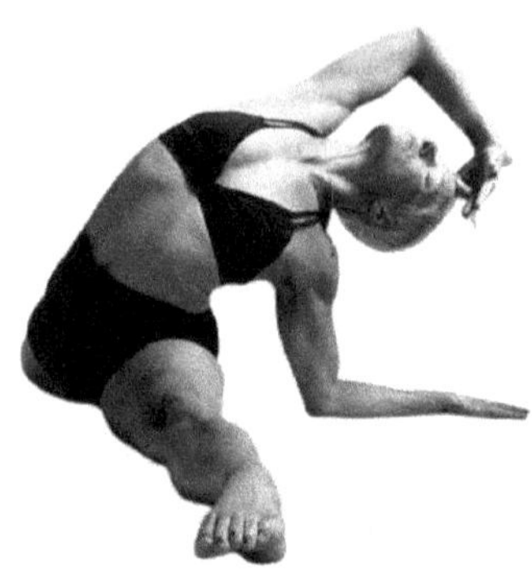

- Sit on the floor with one leg extended and the other bent, placing the sole against the inner thigh of the extended leg.

- Reach towards your toes, holding for 15-30 seconds before switching legs.

7. **Seated Forward Bend**:

- Seated with legs extended, hinge at the hips, and reach forward towards your toes.

- Hold for 15-30 seconds, feeling the stretch along your hamstrings and lower back.

8. *Inner Thigh Stretch*:

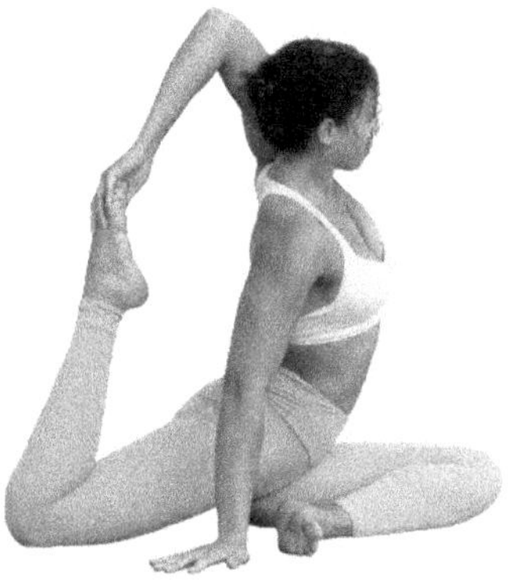

- Sit with legs wide apart, leaning to one side and reaching toward your toes.

- Hold for 15-30 seconds before leaning to the opposite side.

9. **Hip Flexor Stretch**:

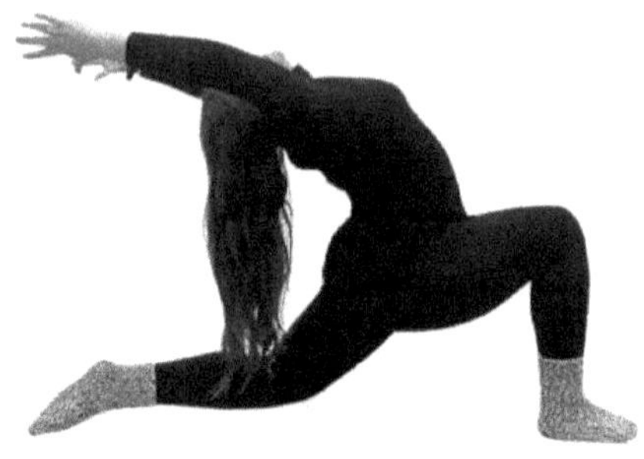

- Kneel on one knee with the other foot in front, forming a 90-degree angle.

- Lean forward, stretching the hip of the kneeling leg.

- Hold for 15-30 seconds, then switch sides.

10. **Cool Down**:

- Conclude your routine with a cool-down, incorporating slow walking or gentle static stretches to gradually bring your heart rate and breathing back to normal.

Always be attentive to your body's signals, refrain from bouncing during stretches, and seek advice from a healthcare professional before commencing a new exercise regimen, especially if you have pre-existing health conditions.

"Stretching is not
a competition or a
chore, but a way
to enhance your
health and
happiness."

CHAPTER 4:

How to Customize Your Stretching Routine

1. *Evaluate Your Requirements*:
Assess which areas of your body require attention, whether it's addressing tightness in specific muscles or aiming for overall flexibility.

2. *Establish Clear Objectives*:
Define your stretching goals, be it enhancing flexibility, alleviating muscle tension, or expanding your range of motion. Clearly outlined objectives will shape your customization approach.

3. *Integrate Targeted Stretches*:
Customize your routine by including stretches that specifically target the identified areas of concern. For instance, if prolonged sitting is a concern, incorporate stretches that focus on opening the hips.

4. *Adjust Duration and Frequency*:
Modify the duration and frequency of your routine based on your schedule and fitness level.

Consistency matters, so find a suitable rhythm, whether it's a daily commitment or multiple sessions per week.

5. ***Dynamic vs. Static Stretches***:
Tailor the combination of dynamic and static stretches in your routine. Dynamic stretches work well for warm-ups, while static stretches contribute to improved flexibility. Strike a balance that suits your personalized needs.

6. ***Listen to Your Body***:
Be attuned to your body's responses during stretches. If you encounter pain (distinct from discomfort), tweak the intensity or seek guidance from a professional.

7. ***Embrace Variety***:
 Keep your routine engaging by incorporating a diverse range of stretches. This not only prevents monotony but also ensures a holistic stretch for various muscle groups.

8. ***Combine with Complementary Exercises:***
 Merge stretching with other exercise forms like yoga or strength training. This synergy enhances overall fitness and flexibility.

9. ***Utilize Props or Supports***:
Personalize your routine by integrating props or aids such as yoga blocks or resistance bands. These tools can facilitate deeper stretches and target specific muscles.

10. ***Regularly Reevaluate***:
Periodically reassess your stretching routine. Adjustments are essential as your flexibility improves or your goals evolve, ensuring your routine remains aligned with your changing needs.

Remember, customization is the cornerstone of an effective stretching routine, tailored to your unique goals, preferences, and body responses.

4.1 How to Incorporate Stretching into Your Daily Activities

1. **Morning Wake-Up Stretch**:

Begin your day with a gentle stretching routine. Extend your body towards the sky and then lean forward at the waist. This helps awaken your muscles and boost flexibility.

2. **Desk Stretches at Work:**

If you're desk-bound, take short breaks for stretching. Perform seated stretches for your neck, shoulders, and wrists. Stand up and stretch your legs and back to counteract the effects of prolonged sitting.

3. **Stretching Breaks**:

Infuse brief stretching breaks into your day. Set a timer to prompt standing up and stretching your arms, legs, and spine. These short intervals prevent stiffness and enhance circulation.

4. **Evening Relaxation Stretch**:

Unwind in the evening with soothing stretches. Concentrate on areas that accumulate tension, like your neck, shoulders, and lower back.

Consider incorporating gentle yoga poses for added relaxation.

5. **Incorporate Stretching in Daily Tasks**:

Blend stretching into your daily routine. While brushing your teeth, waiting for coffee, or standing in line, perform simple stretches such as calf raises, ankle circles, or side bends.

6. **Stretching Before Bed**:

Include a brief stretching routine before bedtime. Gentle stretches for your entire body can promote muscle relaxation, contribute to better sleep, and enhance overall flexibility.

7. **Outdoor Stretching**:

Utilize outdoor spaces for stretching. If you have a garden or access to a park, integrate stretching into your outdoor activities. Enjoy the fresh air while engaging in stretches targeting different muscle groups.

8. **Family Stretching Time**:

Turn stretching into a family activity. Gather everyone for a few minutes of group stretching. This not only fosters physical well-being but also creates a positive shared experience.

9. **Mindful Stretching**:

Practice mindful stretching. Focus on your body and breath during stretches. This not only amplifies the physical benefits but also provides a mental break, reducing stress.

10. **Consistency is Key**:

Maintain a consistent stretching routine. Whether it's a brief morning session or a longer evening stretch, regularity is essential for reaping the full advantages of stretching.

Remember to be attuned to your body, adjust stretches as necessary, and consult a healthcare professional if you have concerns or underlying health conditions.

4.2 How to Use Props to Enhance Your Stretching Experience

Recognize the advantages of integrating props into your stretching regimen. Props can amplify stretches, boost flexibility, and enhance overall comfort throughout your exercises.

- **Yoga Strap for Enhanced Flexibility:**

Employ a yoga strap to elongate your reach in various stretches, especially beneficial for hamstring and shoulder stretches, or any pose requiring increased flexibility.

- **Blocks for Stability:**

Integrate yoga blocks to provide steadiness and support. Position blocks beneath your hands in forward bends or use them to modify poses, ensuring proper alignment and reducing the risk of strain.

- **Bolster for Relaxation:**

Include a bolster, particularly in restorative stretches. Placing a bolster beneath your spine or knees can add comfort and relaxation, fostering ease during prolonged holds.

- **Exercise Ball for Core Engagement:**

Utilize an exercise ball to activate your core during stretching. Incorporate the ball in balance exercises or as support in backbends, intensifying the challenge and effectiveness of your stretches.

- **Foam Roller for Myofascial Release:**

Integrate a foam roller for releasing muscle tension. Glide the foam roller along different muscle groups to encourage myofascial release, aiding in muscle recovery and enhancing overall flexibility.

- **Chair for Modified Poses:**

Utilize a chair for modified versions of poses, particularly beneficial for those with limited mobility or seeking a gentler approach. Chairs offer additional support and stability.

- **Theraband for Resistance:**

Use a Theraband to introduce resistance to your stretches. Incorporate it into arm or leg stretches to intensify muscle engagement, simultaneously promoting strength and flexibility.

- ### Mindful Breathing with Props:

Combine props with mindful breathing techniques. Sync your breath with stretches to deepen relaxation and foster a connection between mind and body.

- ### Closing Thoughts:

Reflect on how incorporating props into your stretching routine can customize and optimize your experience. Experiment with different props to discover what suits your body and individual requirements.

Remember to commence gradually, heed your body's signals, and seek advice from a fitness professional if you have specific health considerations or concerns.

" The more you stretch,
the more benefits you will
reap. Aim to stretch at
least 3 times a week,
preferably every day, and
vary your stretches to
target different muscles
and joints."

CHAPTER 5:

How to Deal with Common Challenges or Obstacles

1. **Identifying Challenges**:
Start by recognizing typical hurdles linked to stretching exercises, such as muscle stiffness, limited flexibility, or discomfort in specific areas.

2. **Gradual Progression**:
Avoid rapid advancements in intensity and duration. Progress gradually to allow your body to adapt, reducing the risk of injury.

3. **Modify Exercises**:
If a specific stretch proves challenging, consider adapting it. Use props or adjust the range of motion to make exercises more manageable while retaining their benefits.

4. **Listen to Your Body**:

Be attentive to your body's signals. If you feel pain (not just discomfort), ease off the stretch, and consult with a healthcare professional if necessary.

5. **Consistency is Key**:

Overcoming challenges requires a consistent approach. Stick to your stretching routine, and improvements in flexibility and comfort will come with time.

6. **Seek Professional Guidance**:

If persistent challenges arise, consider seeking advice from a fitness professional or physical therapist. They can offer personalized guidance and exercises to address specific issues.

7. **Mix Up Your Routine**:

Combat monotony by incorporating a variety of stretching exercises targeting different muscle groups to maintain interest.

8. **Patience and Persistence**:

Acknowledge that progress takes time. Exercise patience and persist in your efforts, celebrating small achievements along the way.

9. **Stay Hydrated**:

Proper hydration is essential for muscle function and flexibility. Ensure you drink enough water throughout the day to support your stretching endeavors.

10. **Rest and Recovery**:
Allow your body sufficient rest and recovery time. Muscles need time to repair and adapt, so avoid overtraining and prioritize adequate sleep.

Remember, each person may encounter unique challenges, so tailor these strategies to your specific circumstances. If challenges persist or worsen, consulting with a healthcare professional is advisable.

5.1 How to Measure Your Progress and Celebrate Your Achievements

- **Establish Clear Objectives:**
Commence by defining specific and attainable goals for your stretching routine. Whether it involves enhancing flexibility, alleviating discomfort, or achieving specific stretch durations, having distinct objectives provides guidance.

- **Record Your Initial State:**
Document your starting capabilities and flexibility levels. This serves as a reference point for comparison as you advance.

- **Consistent Tracking:**
Maintain a regular log of your stretching sessions, noting the duration, types of stretches, and any variations. Consistent tracking helps identify trends and areas for improvement.

- **Utilize Visual References:**
Consider capturing photos or videos of your stretching sessions. Visual documentation can effectively showcase progress over time.

- **Quantify Flexibility:**

Periodically reassess your flexibility using precise measurements. This may involve reaching for your toes, assessing range of motion, or other relevant metrics.

- **Evaluate Comfort Levels**:
Pay attention to your body's sensations during and after stretching. Reduced discomfort or increased comfort in specific stretches signifies progress.

- **Acknowledge Small Achievements**:
Recognize and celebrate minor successes throughout your journey. Whether it's extending a stretch for a few extra seconds or experiencing improved flexibility, every accomplishment matters.

- **Establish Milestones**:
Break down overarching goals into smaller, achievable milestones. Reaching these milestones fosters a sense of accomplishment and motivates ongoing effort.

- **Share Progress**:
Share your progress with friends, family, or a supportive community. External encouragement can amplify your motivation.

- **Reward Yourself**:

When reaching significant milestones, treat yourself to a reward. This could be a small indulgence, a modest purchase, or any form of self-appreciation.

- **Reflect on Achievements**:

Take moments to reflect on your journey's progress. Appreciate the distance covered and acknowledge the dedication invested.

- **Adjust Goals Appropriately**:

Periodically reassess your overall fitness objectives. As you attain milestones, modify and establish new challenges to sustain continuous progress.

Remember, your progress is a personal voyage, and celebrating achievements, regardless of their scale, contributes to a positive and motivating fitness experience.

CONCLUSION

This "Stretching Exercises for Seniors Over 60" transcends being a mere guide; it stands as a testimony to the profound impact of incorporating straightforward yet impactful stretches into your daily life. Throughout our exploration of these tailored exercises, a consistent theme emerged—an invitation to embrace a renewed sense of well-being through empowered movement.

For seniors, each stretch serves as a stride towards heightened flexibility, enhanced balance, and a revitalized overall health. Beyond the physical advantages, this book advocates for a mindful connection with one's body, promoting a seamless integration of movement into the graceful aging process.

As you engage with the techniques outlined in these pages, recognize that this isn't just about adhering to a fitness routine; it's a journey toward reclaiming vitality. The incremental advancements, the celebration of milestones, and the recognition of personal achievements all contribute to a comprehensive approach to senior well-being.

In the tapestry of aging gracefully, these stretches emerge as threads of resilience, weaving a narrative of strength, adaptability, and an indomitable spirit that characterizes the golden years. It's an open invitation to appreciate each stretch, revel in newfound agility, and delight in the progress towards a more dynamic and satisfying life.

May these stretching exercises not only add longevity to your years but infuse life with vitality. Embrace the movements, relish in the achievements, and take joy in the pursuit of an active lifestyle—proving that age is a mere number, and the most fulfilling stretches of life can be experienced at any phase. Here's to a happier, healthier, and more flexible you!.

Dive into the next page to get the journal and Self reflection Question prompt that will improve you!.

DATE: ....

DAILY EXERCISES

HOW DO YOU FEEL TODAY AFTER YOUR EXERCISE

LIST OF TODAY EXERCISES:

Overall time used

TODAY APPRECIATION

What motivated you to start incorporating stretching exercises into your routine, and have those motivations evolved over time?

DATE: ....

DAILY EXERCISES

HOW DO YOU FEEL TODAY AFTER YOUR EXERCISE

LIST OF TODAY EXERCISES:

Overall time used

TODAY APPRECIATION

How has the journey of incorporating stretching exercises impacted your overall sense of well-being and daily life?

DATE: ....

DAILY EXERCISES

HOW DO YOU FEEL TODAY AFTER YOUR EXERCISE

LIST OF TODAY EXERCISES:

Overall time used

TODAY APPRECIATION

As you progressed through the stretching routine, what physical and mental changes did you observe?

DATE: ....

S M T W T F S

⚘ DAILY EXERCISES ⚘

HOW DO YOU FEEL TODAY AFTER YOUR EXERCISE

LIST OF TODAY EXERCISES:

Overall time used

TODAY APPRECIATION

Which specific stretches or exercises resonated with you the most, and why?

DATE: ....

DAILY EXERCISES

HOW DO YOU FEEL TODAY AFTER YOUR EXERCISE

LIST OF TODAY EXERCISES:

Overall time used

TODAY APPRECIATION

Have you shared your stretching journey with others? How has community or social support played a role in your experience?

DATE: ....

DAILY EXERCISES

HOW DO YOU FEEL TODAY AFTER YOUR EXERCISE

LIST OF TODAY EXERCISES:

Overall time used

TODAY APPRECIATION

Reflect on the challenges you encountered during the stretching journey. How did you overcome them, and what did you learn in the process?

DATE: ....

S M T W T F S
○ ○ ○ ○ ○ ○ ○

🏃 DAILY EXERCISES 🏃

HOW DO YOU FEEL TODAY AFTER YOUR EXERCISE

____

____

____

____

LIST OF TODAY EXERCISES:

____

____

____

____

____

Overall time used

TODAY APPRECIATION

____

____

____

In what ways has the book influenced your understanding of the connection between movement, mindfulness, and aging gracefully?

Consider any unexpected or surprising discoveries you made during your stretching journey. How did these revelations influence your perspective on aging and fitness?

DATE: ....

🏃 DAILY EXERCISES 🏃

HOW DO YOU FEEL TODAY AFTER YOUR EXERCISE

LIST OF TODAY EXERCISES:

Overall time used

TODAY APPRECIATION

DATE: ....

DAILY EXERCISES

HOW DO YOU FEEL TODAY AFTER YOUR EXERCISE

LIST OF TODAY EXERCISES:

Overall time used

TODAY APPRECIATION

Think about the impact of stretching on your daily activities. How has increased flexibility and mobility affected your daily life and functional movements?

Consider the milestones you've achieved in your stretching practice. How did you celebrate these achievements, and what further goals do you aspire to reach?

S M T W T F S
○ ○ ○ ○ ○ ○ ○

DAILY EXERCISES

HOW DO YOU FEEL TODAY AFTER YOUR EXERCISE

LIST OF TODAY EXERCISES:

Overall time used

TODAY APPRECIATION